FOCUSED MEDITATION

THE ORDERLY CONTROL OF THE MIND TO UNLOCK CREATIVITY

From the Author of:

Simon Peter. The making of a man of faith.
Money. Don't settle for less.
Give us this day our daily bread.
Embracing Prosperity.
You will Prosper.
Possessing your Promised Land.
Be the Head and Not the Tail.
and
Praying This Way.

Malcolm Baxter
MIFS DipFA CISI CertPFS

First published in Great Britain in 2018
Malcolm Baxter
Aston House
126 Grove Road
Tring
Hertfordshire
HP23 5PA
Malcolm@muchinmind.com
www.muchinmind.com

ISBN: 978-1-9998307-3-1

Published by: GS2 Design Ltd.
www.GS2design.co.uk

Index

Acknowledgements

I am grateful to the support of my longsuffering wife Margaret during the writing of this book. It took only a few days to write, much longer to edit and years to practise, experience and refine, into a readable product. She knows it all even without needing to read it herself!

To the many literary scholars, sages, mystics and skilled writers through the ages who have discovered for themselves first and then recorded, the truths which have instructed me. They are my mentors, counselors and guides.

To the members of the Prosperity Academy, who attend my courses, and to whom I deliver 'what I have just found out'. Their support and continued attendance keep me focused on moving them forward on this remarkable journey of discovery.

To Pastor Wendy, who never stops encouraging me, and confirming to me that I 'have something' which needs to be told.

To Graham who has designed all the printed matter, DVDs, CDs marketing material and fliers. *It looks great.*

Malcolm Baxter
www.muchinmind.com

Malcolm Baxter

Introduction

Focused Meditation
The orderly control of the mind to unlock creativity

Focused Meditation is the orderly control of the mind to unlock creativity.

There are four distinct stages comprising a process which, if applied carefully, will undoubtedly bring great success.

These stages are: self-awareness, forming the desire, visualisation and affirmation.

Whenever we imagine things as they ought to be rather than as they seem to be, we establish a creative moment. Nothing could be more important to anyone. This is the key to transformation in our lives in all respects.

Having been invited to speak at a convention, and having chosen as my subject, 'Focused Meditation', the outline I submitted, caused the committee who selected me to ask for a more in depth presentation. I prepared a further presentation, which covers what I had in mind and in more detail. But I was conscious that I would still only be scratching the surface of what is needed to do justice to the subject.

This subject, or at least the title which I have coined, is so unfamiliar to many that I have been exploring what the words mean by searching Wikipedia, Oxford English Dictionary and The School of Meditation publication 'Being Oneself.'

I conclude that this is not a familiar expression – 'Focused Meditation' – but of course we know what it could refer to. The well known and understood aspect of 'meditation' needs no explanation, and I will not aim to deal with it in detail in this book.

I differentiate Focused Meditation from the originally eastern styles of meditation.

Traditional meditation is one which essentially removes all thoughts from the mind, except to concentrate on something mundane – one's breathing particularly or some aspect of nature, in a still, restful, calm and quiet state. The benefits of this behaviour are for relaxation, peacefulness and inward contemplation and some meditators experience physical healing.

Traditional Meditation will not change the events which befall us in our lives, but it can change the way we react to those events – but it produces little chance of anything new.

F W Whiting, London School of Meditation Handbook "Being Oneself."

By contrast, Focused Meditation uses the dictionary understanding of the word 'meditation' meaning *Plan mentally, design, exercise the mind.* The Greek root, med- means *to think about.*

Therefore, the application of quiet calm and deliberate control of the mind relate to both traditional and focused meditation, but the power of using meditation for a creative purpose is not. Focused Meditation is the creative purpose – which seems to have been hidden from most of us, and not taught in our society.

This book explains and emphasises the control of the mind. It creates a process to follow as the steps to take into easily understood and applied mental disciplines. This will become a lifestyle choice for everyone who desires to be successful.

Three dimensional and four dimensional.

We will also cover the spiritual aspects of what we are considering, because everything we see in this world (or otherwise validate by our five senses) comes from what we cannot see. When we cannot see something which we believe exists, it is a spiritual concept, and is the way we are created and we ourselves create.

The following diagram shows the relationship between the outside life of influence upon each of us, and the inside life of subconscious response to those outside influences.

The mind is referred to as either objective or conscious on the one hand and subjective or subconscious on the other.

The conscious mind is occupied with what can be validated by the use of the five senses. The subconscious mind is spiritual and operates on what cannot be seen, but believed.

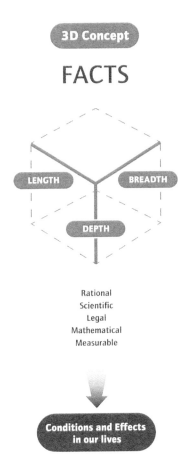

This is the 3 dimensional picture of who we are.

If I were to meet you in the street, the first glance would show me the 3 dimensional you. I can apply the senses of measurement, form, touch, sound and smell. At that stage there will be many physical evidences in the same objective category, which we can measure, feel and smell – visible in the same way that you are.

In that way, much of what we have been taught throughout life is evidenced similarly. We look at a bank statement and read the figures. Or we can boil a kettle on the stove, we can watch the rain fall and we can switch a light on. All this is supported by scientific laws or rules which are immutable. Gravity which we look at by virtue of its effect upon the visible objects around us works continually with measurable precision. Seeing is believing in this world.

Money is particularly interesting, because not only can it be seen in a 3 dimensional way, but also it is there when it cannot be seen. We will cover that later, but certainly we must agree, what we can see is the actual coinage and national treasury notes called currency, and we agree it is competitive money; in a 3 dimensional world – if you have it, I don't; if I have it you don't.

Our 3 dimensional world comprises essentially the facts. The certainty of these facts is always reassuring. Our legal system is based upon provable information. Aeronautics and all scientific processes are quantifiable and consistent.

However, we are spiritual people. For an example, we cannot actually see gravity but we believe in it because we can see the effect it has. We cannot see faith but we use it every day, by working for our wage and believing that we will be paid eventually. These may be just two simple illustrations, but there are many more which will come to mind.

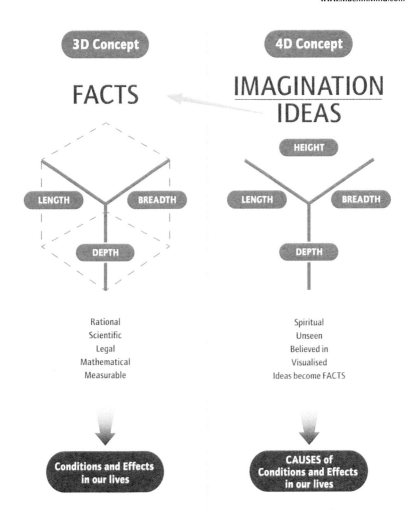

In order to illustrate the 'spiritual' world view, we can describe that unseen element as an additional dimension, the 4th dimension.

It is this 4th dimension which focuses our minds on what we all know about as spiritual, but which many ignore.

Firstly, notice that we carry over the 3D principles of length, depth and breadth, which is a solid form and suggests the cube, but we add height. That represents the spiritual world of what we cannot see. Our subconscious minds find it a problem to have that fourth dimension because it doesn't fit neatly into a shape. But our conscious minds can instruct our subconscious that it is the 'new default' to our responses to the world around us.

We can easily see the tension between the 3D world and the 4D world, because of the uncertainty of being convinced about what we cannot actually see. The 3D world feeds the 4D world with the ultimate material evidence of things, and the 4D world feeds the 3D world with the creation of what will ultimately become visible.

The fourth dimension provides the creativity in ideas and imagination, until they become facts – and materialise.

There is absolutely nothing in our world which has materialised by any other means than imagination in someone's mind. Somebody had to have the idea, and believed it would work. The imagination worked on the idea, and it could then be seen in the mind first. Because our universe is based upon a system of belief in what cannot now be seen, that imagined idea becomes a material fact as a consequence. The universal, natural law says, "whatever you desire, when you pay attention to it, and believe that you already have what you desire, you will have it."

Focused Meditation is the way to put this into parctise, with certain success.

What do you and I desire? If we know what we desire, whatever it is, we can bring it into materialisation. This book will show how by describing what will work for you and me, and the only way to succeed.

Chapter 1

Self Awareness and Understanding
"Who are you? Who am I?"

I AM is a feeling of permanent awareness. I may forget who I am, where I am, what I am, but I cannot forget that I AM. It is my concept of myself in my reactions to life which determines the world in which I live. In other words, if I am experiencing financial limitation, the cause is nothing other than my reactions to life, as a result of my self awareness, and I define this self image by saying "I AM poor." If I assume a different concept of self and rearrange the I AM to "I AM rich," then this will come true.

"Whether you think you can or think you can't,
either way you are right." – *Henry Ford*

We obviously know the 3D understanding of who we are, and we will be certain of our conscious mind also. The conscious understanding relates to what we can see in ourselves – our own self-consciousness.

We can evaluate our personality, our likes and dislikes, our natural gifts and abilities, attributes and beliefs.

But what is so much more difficult for us to truly assess is the 4D aspect of who we are. In this I am saying that the spiritual world is partly evident in those attributes and beliefs we acknowledge, but what we also have is conditioning. Behind those attributes and beliefs is the answer to the question "Why?" Why am I who I think I am?

We understand this question "why I am what I think I am" when you and I realise there is much of our subconscious which has been conditioned by the world around us, and which we have imbibed since our earliest moments of life. Conditioning to life has come from parents, education, peer-group, friends and associates, and from our own studies and determination. Conditioning has made us who we are.

This gives rise to behaviour which is unique to ourselves, but is similar to many others who have been influenced in the same way as ourselves. For instance, our political and religious attitudes are naturally conformed to those of our families and peer groups, with whom we have lived. While we may subsequently change our minds, the subconscious will continue to prescribe the automatic behaviour originally appropriate, until our habits and conversation change also. And even that change will invariably need to conform to what others think in order for us to be comfortable with whatever we now agree with.

A perfect illustration of this is with money. And there are many other very significant aspects of conditioning. We often pass off an attitude as 'our opinion', but without challenging, or needing to challenge ourselves as to why and where did we obtain that opinion and conditioning. Examples are health (or the fear of ill health), ageism, fears of water, spiders, heights, etc. and particularly our perception of where we fit in to society; "we know our place." "upstairs or downstairs?"

But for simplicity, we will just deal with money, as a way of challenging ourselves over self evaluation and understanding.

If we contrast our personal views of rich people and poor people, we will immediately see in ourselves, evidences of subconscious conditioning. This conditioning is a major contributor to why we are rich or poor. Most people like you and me don't normally take this into account, because we cannot measure it, and therefore don't believe it exists. But it certainly does exist.

The reason why this is important is because subconscious conditioning is a limitation in our lives. If we are conditioned against money, we will never be prosperous. Similarly, if we are conditioned to accept infirmity in old age, that is what we will get. If we are conditioned to fear being in a car accident, we increase the risk of it happening to us. The reason for all this is that we have been impressed in our developmental stages of life to accept something we heard, something we saw or something we experienced as being an influence which we will always be conditioned by. Our conscious and objective minds have accepted that as the default setting for our reactions to life as we experience it.

Let us go back to money. How would you respond to these statements:

Rich people believe, "I create my life,"
poor people believe "Life just happens to me."

The rich play the money game to win.
The poor people play the money game not to loose.

Rich people are committed to being rich.
Poor people want to be rich.

Rich people focus on opportunities.
Poor people focus on obstacles.

Rich people admire other rich and successful people.
Poor people resent rich and successful people.*

Taken from 'Secrets of the Millionaire Mind', T Harv Eker,

"The mind is everything. What you think, you become." – Buddha

If this is a true statement, then what we have become is what we are right now, and the way in which we became what we are right now is as a result of the thoughts we have had in our heads. We cannot blame outside influences and conditioning – they were our thoughts we had. The economy, politics, an unhelpful upbringing etc. are all external effects, which have not in themselves made us what we are. It is just what we have been thinking which has made you 'you' and me 'me'.

So if we understand that position we can so easily see that if today we change the way we think, our tomorrow will be different from what it is today. If we don't change our mindset today, tomorrow will look just like today. But all of us want a different tomorrow, in some respect, so we now know what to do, and we now know it will work.

"All power is from within and therefore under our control."
– Robert Collier "The Secret of The Ages"

In order for us to be able to control our minds, so that we focus our meditation, we need to deal with our conditioning, in relation to what is our desire. If we desire more money, then we firstly need to confirm that we are rich people now.

"When someone becomes a millionaire, the least important thing is what they have. The most important thing is what they have become." – Malcolm Baxter

Just looking at those contrasts is a challenge to each of us, because we naturally want to put ourselves in one of the two categories. Either we are conditioned to be rich, and are therefore comfortable with that status in life, or we are not rich, and would be uncomfortable to be rich, in some way.

The good news is that if we are not rich, then provided we alter our thinking we can be. The suggestions in the contrasts are that there are specific reasons why we may have conditioning which works against us. For instance in the first one, we know that rich people are characterised as those who take authority over what affects them and 'get their own way.' Poor people are those who do the opposite. They blame others around them, the economy, their unfulfilling job, political uncertainty and even the person they married; but never themselves.

If you or I fall into the poor category it is because we have imbibed the values and opinions of other people, and adopted their philosophy on life. But a change of mind will open the doors to re-educating the subconscious to accept a rich mindset. To reach a higher level of being, you and I must assume a higher concept of ourselves. If you and I will not imagine ourselves as other than what we are, then we will remain as we are.

For anyone unfamiliar with the book quoted here by T Harv Eker, it is one I would recommend you read. The book clearly shows us that if we have a poor person mindset, we are hindering prosperity – it will not come anywhere near you or me.

Focused Meditation allows space to adjust the thinking, and make sure that it is used to clear away the hindrances of wrong thinking inherited from the past. There is no way the universe will give you or I abundant wealth if we have anything against wealthy people. Also, if we were to curse money by saying words like, "I can't afford it," or "I'm never paid enough" that lack of gratitude will stop the universe from answering your desire for more money. Similarly, if we are ill, the universe will not bring us healing if we complain about the health service, doctors, medication, or indeed complain about the condition itself. And some want more clients in their business, so if they complain about not enough good clients and doing services which they are not wanting to do or don't get paid enough to do, the universe will not give us anything other than that. Measure everything against the standard of 'gratitude for what we have now.'

So we meditate upon the positive only as a new default position for our meditation, and we understand ourselves, and the prosperity which we now attract.

Chapter 2

Forming Desires

Someone once said, "The reason why people don't get what they want is because they don't know what they want." Is that a true statement?

The truth is that the law of the universe is immutable in that we always get what we desire – always without fail. Remarkably to some, that law does not fail for a moment – it is, after all, a law of the universe. How could a natural universal law fail to work?

So, if someone complains, "I never get what I want," we must know that they got their desire, but it was not what they wanted. How did that happen? They will always get what they desired, but it may not be what was good for them.

The universe will never discriminate for you and me what is good for us, nor for what is bad for us. We have the total right of freedom in the choices we make. The universe only gives us what we are paying attention to as a desire. If it is bad for us, then it has just as much right to turn up in our lives as if it is good for us. The law works as we tell it to. If you or I decide to be poor, then that is what turns up. If we decide to be rich, then that will turn up. As the difference is entirely the result of what we have thought, and paid attention to, it is totally within our control to get what is good for us, all of the time.

Focused Meditation is the way we can take time out to contemplate on what is good for us, and eliminate thoughts and feeling which are contrary to those desires we have.

This book is just laying the foundations for right thinking, so don't give up reading it. We are considering the orderly control of the mind to unlock creativity.

I like the word 'desire' because it is a powerful word. The OED tells us that it means 'longing for' or 'craving for.' There is an ambition about this; it is out of the ordinary. It is a dominant feeling. The word is used in the Bible when Jesus summarises the law of the universe so succinctly "Whatever you desire, when you pay it attention, believe that you have it already and it will be yours."

We all fill our minds with wishes and hopes. We are also inclined to hold fears and doubts in our minds. Out of that maelstrom of mental activity, which goes on all the time, Focused Meditation is required to pick out the hopes and dreams of what we want, and get rid of the fears and doubts. It takes time and persistence.

If you and I don't do that we will find that we thought of something we wanted and attached to that thought was the fear. "I can't afford it," "What will people think?" and so on. Probably, the fear is what brought the thought to mind, particularly if it was about money. The universe will be confused because the negative and the positive appear together, and therefore nothing happens. Fear will always cancel out the positive.

Many people stumble over this with their health conditions. Perhaps the thought comes into their mind, "I am in pain this morning." They immediately confirm with their partner that they need sympathy because of the pain. And then they may hope that it is better soon, but they go to the Doctor to confirm they are in pain and want to be cured. The doctor agrees that they are in pain, and to have a pain in this place could be serious enough to warrant a second opinion. And so the process escalates. The pain gets worse, and more and more people are involved to bolster the negative belief.

In that scenario, the attention was being paid to the negative condition, and it was believed in. Faith in the continuing and worsening pain was followed by works which agreed with the pain and confirmed by words spoken about it. The universe would conclude that the person in pain wanted more pain. And that is what happens – more pain.

Such a person's desire is in reverse. They will get what they don't want and not what they do want. But if we understand that situation, because it is only life as we know it, then suppose we turn it round and have a desire which has the same commitment and craving, but expressed in a positive way for something which would be good for us. If we want money for instance, firstly, when the desire comes to mind, we must tear off the fear tag of 'not enough' and replace it with a feeling of plenty, and a spirit of thanksgiving for all we have. Say the affirmation, "The universe will supply all my needs out of its abundance, and everything I receive I bless." We don't go around seeking sympathy from others over our limited circumstances, but are happy that the promise of abundance has already materialised.

So the formulation of the desire, is to commit ourselves to really wanting it with all our hearts. A casual hope or wish will inevitably have a negative thought attached, which cancels it out. We must feel our desire to be intense and dominant.

For Focused Meditation, the concept of imagination is vital, because this desire is for something which cannot be seen at the present time. It is only in the mind. At this stage, we have decided that it is what we really want, and we will do whatever we need to get it.

So what I do is I write it down. I have a Journal which I write in every day, and one aspect is that I describe what I desire. The writing of it down embeds the wish to make it into a desire, and it also captures the 'frame' as a 'still', so that I can revert to it and read what I wrote initially; I can confirm that it still is my earnest desire.

In my Focused Meditation, I have my Journal with my desires written there. I tick off the ones which have materialised and retain those which are still outstanding. I normally have about 8 'on the go' but I focus on only one at a time. I select the one which I am most committed to when I focus my meditation.

The whole process of Focused Meditation is to imagine what the future looks like. The desire is what you will have when your future arrives. What does it look like? How does it feel to have it already? The desire could be anything at all. It may be for something big, or small. It is the imagination which will bring it out into the open to allow you to pay it attention.

Not many people are imaginative into the future. The images they have in their minds are memories, and often unhappy. Focused Meditation contemplates now, on what we want for tomorrow, and without imagining it, it will never happen. Please read this example of the power of the imagination:

In 1898, an author, who was not well known called Morgan Robertson, wrote a fictionary story about a fabulous Atlantic Liner, considerably larger than had ever been built before. Robertson described the smug and very rich people who happily set sail in this ship. He also described how on a cold April night it was wrecked on an iceberg, 400 miles from Newfoundland. The book is called "Futility", and was published by the firm of M F Mansfield.

Fourteen years later the British shipping company "White Star Line" built a liner very much like the one in Morgan Robertson's story. The new liner displaced 66,000 tons, Robertson's 45,000 tons. The new ship was 882 feet long, the fictionary one, 800 feet long. They could both carry 3,000 passengers, both could travel at 25 knots, both had three propellers and they both had not enough lifeboats, but as they were both 'unsinkable' it did not matter.

On April 19th, 1912, the real ship left Southampton on her maiden voyage to New York, and she struck an iceberg and sank 400 miles from Newfoundland.

Robertson called his ship "Titan." The White Star Line called its ship, "Titanic."

Of course I would not suggest that Morgan Robertson should take personal responsibility for what happened to the Titanic, but it serves to confirm that imagination is powerful, both negatively and positively. If we can use this awesome power positively for our benefit, and not our detriment, then we certainly do have all we need from within.

Imagination is the cause of everything. It is the creative force in the world. The formulation of your desire starts that creative process. We can imagine the past and it will root us in the past. That will keep on coming back into our present and prevent our progress. But imagining the details of what we want in the future will be the basis for what actually happens. It must become compelling and urgent for us to overcome the negative and fearful thoughts which we find pop up in our minds. Focused Meditation is where all this battlefield of the mind takes place.

Chapter 3

Visualisation

Perhaps the most important element of the entire process of Focused Meditation rests on the 'feeling of the dream fulfilled.'

"We only have to concentrate on the state desired in order to mentally see it. But to give it reality so that it will become an objective fact, we must focus attention on the invisible state until it has the feeling of reality. Only then will we have given it the right to become a visible concrete fact."

— *Neville Goddard*

In the previous chapter we considered about the 'desire.' We emphasised the fact that this needs to be compelling and earnest. We also indicated that it must be consistent and in detail. I suggested the use of a Journal in which to write it down, as an aid to consistency and a trigger to the memory.

Now, in this chapter we deal with that aspect of Focused Meditation which turns that desire into materialisation. The method is visualisation.

Visualisation and imagination are interchangeable words, except that the force of visualisation is consistent with dwelling on the image until it materialises. It is to call up the picture imaged into reality; calling what isn't as if it is. As Robert Collier says:

See things as you would have them be rather than as they are.

The purpose of visualisation is to draw into our minds and our thinking those things that relate to our anticipated lives. We read of being transformed by the renewing of our minds. If we are unaware of being transformed by a renewing process in our minds, then it has not happened. We are still conscious only of being in a 3D world, and the imagined new world available to us by the accurate and conscious use of our imagination is not yet our experience.

Without that revelation, we only see things as they are. The size of our business, the amount we earn, the house we occupy, the kind of car we drive etc. We just see these things as what they are. Yesterday looked just the same, and we expect that tomorrow will also look just the same.

We could struggle with that concept and argue that we are making progress. Good. We should be just because we are alive! That's nothing to shout about! So the principle is validated by a small incremental benefit only.

But is that what you and I want to settle for? Perhaps not. Rich people think big. Poor people look up to rich people. Who are you and I looking up to? Is that what you want to be yourself?

Visualisation is the way in which we change the mind-set so that we are able to bring different results into our lives. We aim to be the people that others look up to. How does that feel?

The importance of feeling the dream fulfilled is fundamental to success. This feeling accepts only that you have already got what you desire, but before you have it. The concept is 'coming from the end' rather than 'towards the end.' If we visualise towards the end as if we are wanting the result while we do not yet have it, we are always visualising not yet having our desire, and so we will remain in the state of not yet having it. But if we come from the feeling of now having our result, then we give the materialisation the right to appear. Feeling is the key. Do we feel we have it or do we feel that we do not have it? That feels completely opposite.

So Focused Meditation concentrates on the feeling of having it already. The temptation is to concentrate on how it will come to you or me. But to concentrate on that means, whatever we say, that we do not believe we have it already. To take into our visualisation the process of how it will come will always keep us in the state of not receiving it – ever.

In the visualisation, imagine having it. Paint the imaginary picture of the new life. Concentrate on the feelings. Bring all the senses into the picture, and experience what you see, hear, taste, smell and particularly how it feels and how you feel in that new life.

When the details of this experience which you imagine are clearly defined, then put movement and people into it. Perhaps you are entertaining friends in your new home. How does your new home feel to you, through their eyes? Do they express words of congratulation? Are you celebrating with them? What are you drinking? While much of that is mundane detail, nevertheless, to feel from the end result means that those observations are there. Feel them. Believe they exist and that those things happen, and they make you feel happy.

The good feeling is now what you are grateful for. We need to cement the visualisation with thankfulness. Giving thanks for something before it actually exists creates a vacuum in the universe, which needs to be filled. Because you said "thank you", what you gave thanks for had to turn up for you in order to validate your gratitude.

Remembering the visualisation is also vital. It may be some time before the desire materialises, so you will go back to it whenever it comes to mind, and particularly during Focused Meditation. The detail needs to be the same, and there should be aspects of the image which will come back repeatedly. Those details are an anchor to your visualisation, and just a flash in the mind of colour, smell, an action or particularly some words said, will bring the whole visualisation back in a fleeting moment.

It may help to note in your Journal some items which trigger the whole visualisation. When materialisation does actually occur, you will find that it seems like the dream was actually the reality, because there is so much the same between the visualisation and the materialisation and the details are often very close to the reality. It is very much like the Titan and the Titanic.

When Margaret and I were considering buying the house we now live in, we had viewed it, and wanted to buy it. The owner agreed to sell it to us but not immediately because he was waiting for the completion of a house which was being built for him. We did not have the money to buy at that time but believed we would have in due course.

The availability of funds was not a certainty – only a belief at that time. So we developed the visualisation along the lines of living in the house. I bought magazines like Ideal Home and House Beautiful which I read from cover to cover in order for me to visualise the new house with our new furniture in it and the colour schemes of our choice. We lived in our imaginations in the house, enjoying entertaining, furnishing the rooms, cooking in the kitchen, drawing our curtains at night. We decided where the grandchildren would sleep when they visited, and the colour choices for those rooms were suited to them. We purchased a few items for the house as corresponding actions of our faith. After six months, the money was received, the house we were buying became vacant, we bought it and we moved in.

The desire we had for that place to live was graphically imagined before it happened. The feeling of actually living in it and enjoying every detail was vital to the integrity of the visualisation. And so the time scale and the synchronisation of the events were so smooth we had to check to make sure it was the reality and not still the visualisation.

The definiteness of the visualisation is crucial. During Focused Meditation we should feed our minds on the detail and the feeling of the fulfillment actually enjoyed; and avoid changing our mind.

You and I must not limit the visualisation to what we think is possible. Remember, you and I have been conditioned by false limitations and limited ambitions during your lives, that is why we are where we now are. The universe is without limits so we go wild and imagine really big. And whenever we convince ourselves of the possibility of something very significant, always add "or something even better." By using the imagination for this activity there is no reason to be limited. The imagination can take us absolutely anywhere, and should do. The promise is 'whatever.' It means 'whatever.'

Chapter 4

Affirmation

When we say something audibly the ears receive the sound physically, and we hear what we have said. That process presents what we have said to our subconscious minds and conditions us to believe that it is true.

We know this is working because we do it all the time. We express arguments aloud, as a way of getting the belief in what we are saying established within us. We are using the process of developing our subconscious responses to react to external influences. Our subconscious minds have no basis for rational choice over whether it is good or bad, it simply receives what it is given; The conscious mind makes that judgment, but the subconscious merely does what it has been educated to do.

The one problem in this is that re-education of the subconscious mind is not easy nor is it quick. That is what is meant by the concept of transforming ourselves by the renewing of the mind.

We went into detail in the introduction about the conditioning of our minds. We saw there that this is reflecting the whole of our lives so far. Many more elderly people are described as stubborn. People say of them "They will die in the ways." The inference is that change is not easy, and many more mature people just cannot change.

But we want to change. The conditions we now experience in our lives are no longer what we want. We know that there is a better life waiting for us to move into, and we just can't wait. That image before us, which we visualise with fervour and critical commitment, day after day, should now be ours. We give thanks for it before we receive it, but somehow it doesn't happen. Does that ring a bell?

Well, the answer could be that we don't expect it to turn up. And the reason why is because our subconscious is getting in the way.

The problem therefore is that if we consider our life now we must agree that it is the sum total of what we have thought. We have accepted all that conditioning, which has given us this which we have accepted and believed. Our subconscious minds have obeyed every instruction our conscious minds have given, based upon what we have heard, what we have seen and what we have experienced. It is most unwilling to choose a different response now.

The conscious mind has been objective about a new way of thinking; a way without those historically appropriate limitations. But how does the conscious mind now retrain the subconscious mind? I quote from Mohammad Ali (of all people!)

It's the repetitions of affirmations that leads to belief. Once that belief becomes a deep conviction, things begin to happen.
— *Mohammad Ali.*

The greatest boxer of all time (possibly) we all remember as the one who boasted "I am the greatest." I can remember him strutting his stuff when he had beaten his opponent to become champion, with this proud boast. But he only became 'The Greatest' as a result of his determination to be so. It is fitting that it should be him who gave us this quotation.

On the way to being world champion, Ali would have needed to work hard, and no doubt he had many doubts and fears to still. He will have developed Focused Meditation for that accomplishment, and during it all he will have laid claim to his creative genius by repeating the words "I am the greatest."

The affirmation is the way in which the subconscious is re-educated. What we say comes straight from the heart and is creative, and when we say it ourselves, it bypasses our objective mind, and instructs our subjective mind. Often repeating the principles in the form of 'sound words of wisdom' will change what our conditioning has created.

The affirmations we should use will connect us to the new world we want to inhabit. They will be statements which describe the right we have to abundance without limits in all areas of our lives. Perhaps we can read them out of good self help books, or make them up ourselves. Invariably the words we use will appear challenging because they are not based upon the 3D view of life which is normal to us. So to affirm, "I am a millionaire, and everything I touch turns to gold" may sound incorrect according to how our lives look at the moment. But those words are exactly what has been in our visualisation – an image of the life we want.

When we say these words, it may help to do so in private, because to be within earshot may cause others to deride our refusal to tell the truth as they see it. Not everyone understands these principles, and you do not want people dragging you down to their level of unbelief.

I have pages of affirmations, which I draw on continually. When I am in Focused Meditation, very much of the description of my ideal condition will be affirmed by me at that time. What about these:

"The universe will supply all my needs according
to its glorious riches."

"With me is the wisdom of the ages. That wisdom now shows me
how to expand my life and my world now. That wisdom shows me
how to prosper as I help others. That wisdom resolves all situations
which I come up against to my greater good."

"My success and prosperity in all I do today is already certain
and I give thanks for it and bless it to me and the people you
give me to bless."

"This day my mind is renewed by understanding right thinking
and I therefore forbid all thoughts of failure and limitation to
inhabit my mind. Wealth and riches are in my house."

Chapter 5

How to – Focused Meditation

Take time! Relax! Be still – very still.

Concentrate on being gentle and loving to yourself.

Stop trying to "get it" just "let it". Let go of tension and strain. Take heart! The whole universe is on your side for you to achieve. You do succeed. You cannot fail. Absorb the glorious feeling that the whole universe is involved in just you. Be still and know.

In the busyness of our lives, to take time out is not easy. The constant demands upon our time and attention make Focused Meditation an obstacle, and an unwelcome additional effort. We are also up against the sense of failure because we expect not to be as diligent in this as we know we should be. We ooze guilt and remorse!

While we all know that there is no option but to find time, nevertheless, to beat ourselves up about it is totally unproductive. Yes, there are things to do in life, particularly in order to be prosperity minded. The items covered so far in this book covering the steps to be taken, and the care about each of those steps is in itself daunting.

One aspect of attitude which may help us, is to differentiate between 'Habits' and 'Self Discipline'.

Habits are the things we do as a regular process because they are good. We know that to clean our teeth in the morning is a good habit. So is going to work and paying the bills on time. Indeed, our lives are filled with good habits; it's reassuringly ordered and safe.

But self-discipline is something which is imposed upon us because we would be worse off if we did not behave in a controlled way. We control the things we eat and drink, so that our bodies are respected. We control our central heating, to stay warm, but not too warm. We control our spending so as to have enough and to spare at all times.

When we consider the time for Focused Meditation, would we put it in the habit part of our lives, or in the self-discipline part?

Let us not put it in the self-discipline part, because then there is a sense of obligation, which we cannot always meet up to. That will inevitably end in a sense of failure and guilt. Even if we applied our self-discipline most days and achieved something towards what we should be doing, even then we would feel that we have let ourselves down, and of course we believe we have no right to benefit from the process. It is similar to a fitness regime where we should do certain exercises and dietary control, and we are not loosing weight. We feel "Of course I'm not loosing weight, because I am not sufficiently diligent." That is a negative, guilt and fear-ridden feeling which will always impose on us a sense of failure.

So, let us consider what we do as a new habit, because that sounds positive and makes us happy. If we don't stick to the new habit, we can pick it up tomorrow, and we have only missed a day. It doesn't feel so bad, does it?

The sense of habit is very important. Everyone sticks to their habits with 100% discipline. On the other hand, self-discipline is always lacking, and what it is lacking are the good habits.

Habits are natural behavioural requirements for ordered living, and common sense. If we stick to a new habit for 21 days, it will become a permanent change in our behaviour. That is positive and helpful to us. It makes us happy because we are believing in progress and a better life. It is ultimately the habits which count, not the self-discipline.
Successful people have successful habits. Unsuccessful people have unsuccessful habits.

I know that the Journal has been mentioned. The best new habit which we could take on is to write in our Journal every day. In this Journal which you keep, you write about what your ideal life looks like. Every item there projects you forward to a situation where you have your desires, and you are living the better life. The fact that you and I may miss a day, here and there, doesn't change our consciousness of prosperity truth, nor does it undermine our confidence in a friendly universe.

But what a habit of writing in your Journal every day will do is it will establish who runs your life today. You and I will write stuff there which will define our plans and purposes for each day, before it happens.

Without that focus first thing each morning, the mind will be assailed by every random thought swilling around in the ether, and the time you and I will waste during the day, meeting the conditions of other peoples agendas, will mean that, like yesterday, your time was not well spent. So this is the one habit which will change your life from too much futility and tail chasing into creative purpose and fulfilment. Prosperity depends on good habits and not self-discipline.

To be practical about Focused Meditation, we must look at what we need to do. I give myself fifteen minutes in the morning. I will be in a quiet place. I will be comfortable and surrounded by my familiar environment. I metaphorically close the door, which means I am disciplined to keep out everything which is distracting for those few short moments.

Distractions could be noise, people, and things of interest. I often close my eyes for some of the time.

I believe that we can all find that still place of communion within and spiritual contemplation. The stillness of those precious minutes can be extremely deep, and produce a sense of guidance and peace over the day to come. Many good ideas and reassurances come to me at that time.

I use this time to say affirmations of what I am trusting in, for instance
"Divine order takes charge of my life this day and every day."
"All things work together for good for me today."
"I am guided all day long and whatever I do today prospers."
"I am a spiritual magnet drawing to me this day exactly all
I need – things, people and situations, all of which are mine by
right, according to the promises of abundant good for me."
"With me is the wisdom of the ages which shows me how to
expand my life and my world now." I have written these and many other affirmations in my Journal so as to be easily available for me.

I always have my journal, and some of it I complete as I Focus Meditate. In that book I have written my desires, and I select one to focus in now. The Focused Meditation on that desire will either require the imagined description to be created or the details will spring to mind if I have already considered that desire before. I spend time living the life of that imagined desire, as if I had already received it. I generate the happy feeling of the dream fulfilled, and give thanks for its completion. I then move on to another desire, according to the time available.

At the end of my Focused Meditation time, I will write down the day's 'To do Today' list, which, in a very few words will identify perhaps four items of activity I will carry out, and the reasons why they are relevant for my progress.

The defined detail of each imagination is in the mind always. Every day we should bring that back to consciousness, at any time, and remembering the feeling of happiness of the desire fulfilled, say "thank you" and then put it down again. That will only take a moment and this continual reaffirmation of the desire, from the view-point of the fulfilled materialisation will hasten its arrival. In fact, when it actually arrives it will be a non-event, because you are living there already.

In effect then, the habitual Focused Meditation time simply establishes what the focus for the day is, and lays a basis for those moments of re-affirmation as the day progresses. These can and should be deliberate reminders, and should be used as a focus particularly when we are under stress. The happy feeling of a desire fulfilled can be drawn into consciousness at any time, particularly when it is to deal with negative and fearful thoughts and situations.

In my Journal I have a page where I have written my "I AMs." The words I AM are written down the left side of the page, and against each I have written a description of myself, as from the view point of 'how the universe sees me.' As the universe's promises are all 'yes' for me, I can confidently write bold words. For instance "I AM creator of my own life" "I AM wealthy" "I AM grateful" "I AM strong," and many more. By writing these, and then reading them as affirmations, I am re-educating my subconscious mind to accept a new way of understanding. I include these statements in the affirmations I say during my Focused Meditation as a conscious way of reminding myself of the truth, even though the evidence before me might suggest otherwise.

Conclusion

The collection of words and phrases which compile this book only mean something to the reader, who accepts them as written. I could use exactly the same words and phrases and write a completely different book, which may well be readable, but which would give a different message.

So also, when we consider life to us in our world, very many aspects are presented to each of us, in the same, or similar ways. However, it is how we absorb those messages as individuals which will determine how we are conditioned.

In reading this book, you will be able to react to my words and phrases from your conditioned point of view, and you have the right to accept and apply the message or to reject it. You could adapt it or change the bits you don't like to suit you.

However, I would ask you to give it a chance. The fact that it has worked for me, and goes on working for me, is evidence that what I have written is what I believe will be of benefit to you also. As the journey is different for us all, what works for me may not be what is right for you. While I have endeavoured to base what I have said on the way I see the world working, even that is a personal, objective view and who am I to claim to be the final word.

But whatever you think, I believe that this approach is valid for everyone, as I have written it. I encourage each reader to spend time carefully understanding and applying the teaching. I will be very surprised if it doesn't work for you as it has done for me. In fact I know it will work for everyone.

"If life for you is not abundant then that is evidence that you have missed the mark. You now have what you chose but didn't mean to choose what you have."

— *Malcolm Baxter*

"Your level of success will rarely exceed your level of personal development, because success is something you attract by the person you become."

— *Jim Rohn*

Ordinary people believe only in the possible. Extraordinary people visualise not what is possible or probable, but rather what is impossible. And by visualising the impossible, they begin to see it as possible.

— *Cherie Carter-Scott.*

Malcolm Baxter

Much in Mind

Much in Mind is a community of people who wish to grow their lives through the exercise of faith in the natural Spiritual Laws of the Universe, often confirmed by the wisdom contained in the words of Jesus.

Because of the writer's personal need to understand about the way these natural spiritual laws of Prosperity Truth impact him, in order to move forward in his quest for success, he found that he needed to write down his discoveries, reasonings and desires, to clarify what he now believes. Having done so, he has written nine books which are shown on the website and are available to buy.

To write the books has allowed him to develop the arguments and true teachings in his own mind, so that this can be effectively explained to others, and also as a benchmark for him for his own development and growth.

Malcolm Baxter has established a coaching program, "Prosperity Academy" where those interested to apply these principles for themselves can share in a community of like minded seekers.

The next step for the reader will make a huge difference in setting him on track towards prosperity; health, wealth and spiritual wellbeing, and the freedoms that attracts.

Malcolm Baxter